SEA MOSS

WHAT DOES SEA MOSS DO FOR YOU?

Sea moss is a prebiotic for your gut, which allows good bacteria to thrive. it is also filled with fiber, which promotes a healthy colon and gastrointestinal system while removing harmful bacteria. Sea moss can also promote weight loss and improved metabolism.

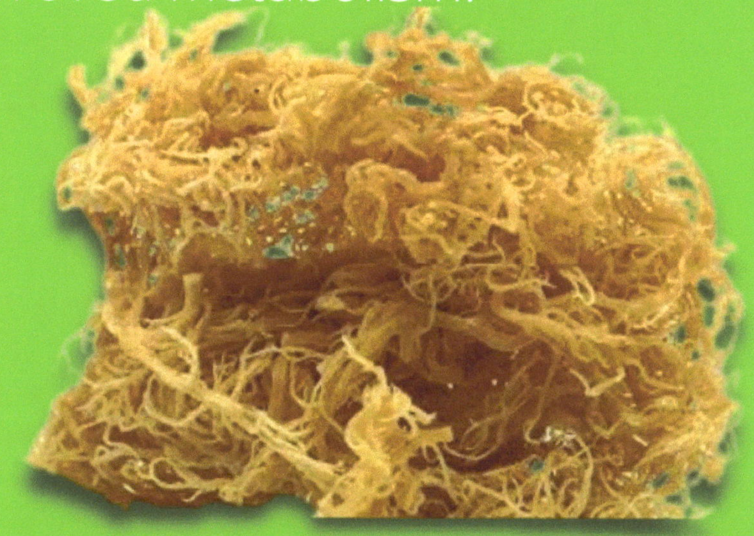

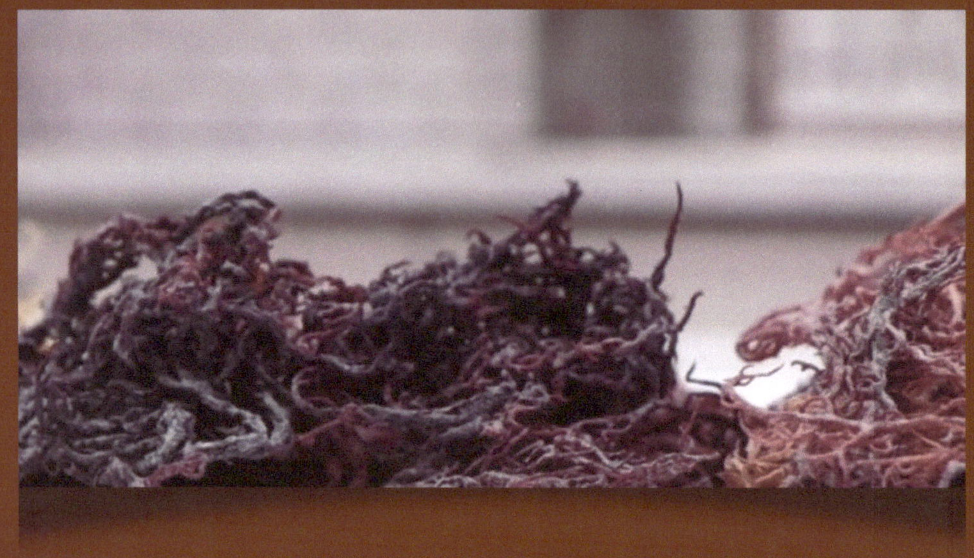

Sea Moss also helps the body fight back against everyday aging and inflammation, in what might be called "the anti's:" Anti-inflammatory, anti-aging, anti-bacterial, and anti-viral. It's used as a treatment to assist prevent and relieve cold and flu-like symptoms, in powdered form.

WHAT ARE THE SIDE EFFECTS OF SEA MOSS?

While it is a good source of iodine, the iodine content of **Sea moss** and other seaweeds are variable. This can put consumers in danger of overconsumption of iodine, which might be problematic. Taking an excessive amount of iodine can cause hypothyroidism or underactive thyroid.

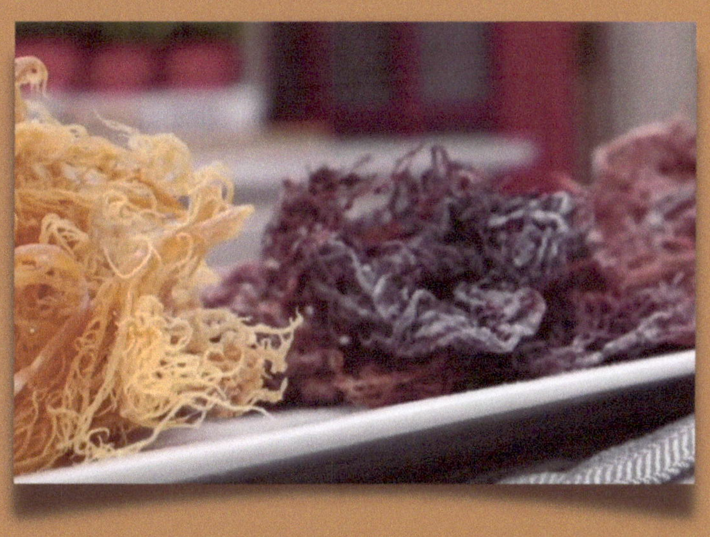

DOES SEA MOSS HELP YOU SEXUALLY?

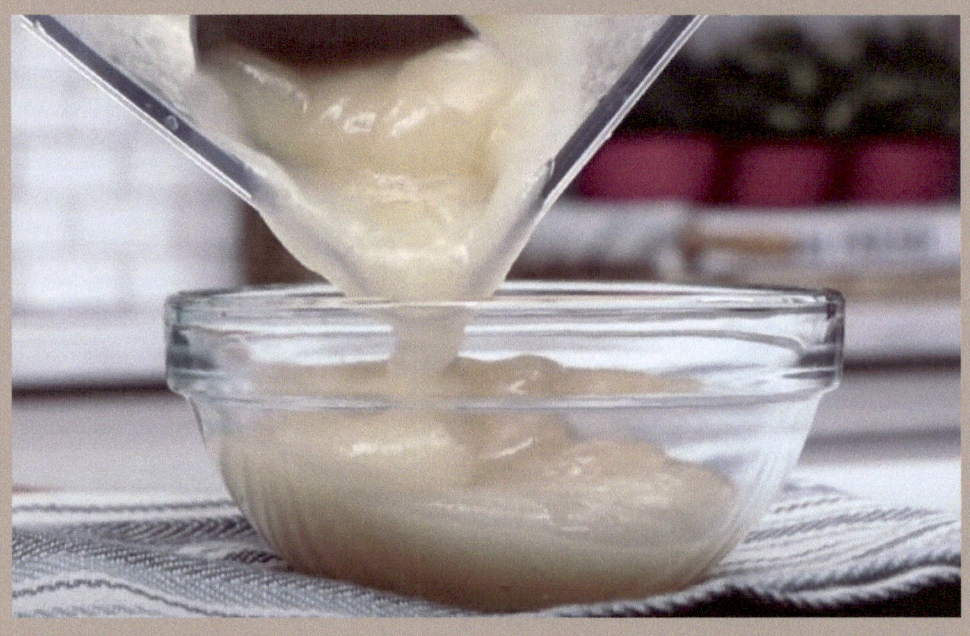

Sea moss is usually used as a natural sexual enhancement product for men in the Caribbean, many say it increases testosterone levels and sperm count, giving fertility a lift.

CAN SEA MOSS HELP WITH WEIGHT LOSS?

Sea moss can increase feelings of fullness, lower body fat, and improve your microbiota profile. It may aid in weight loss due to its carrageenan content.

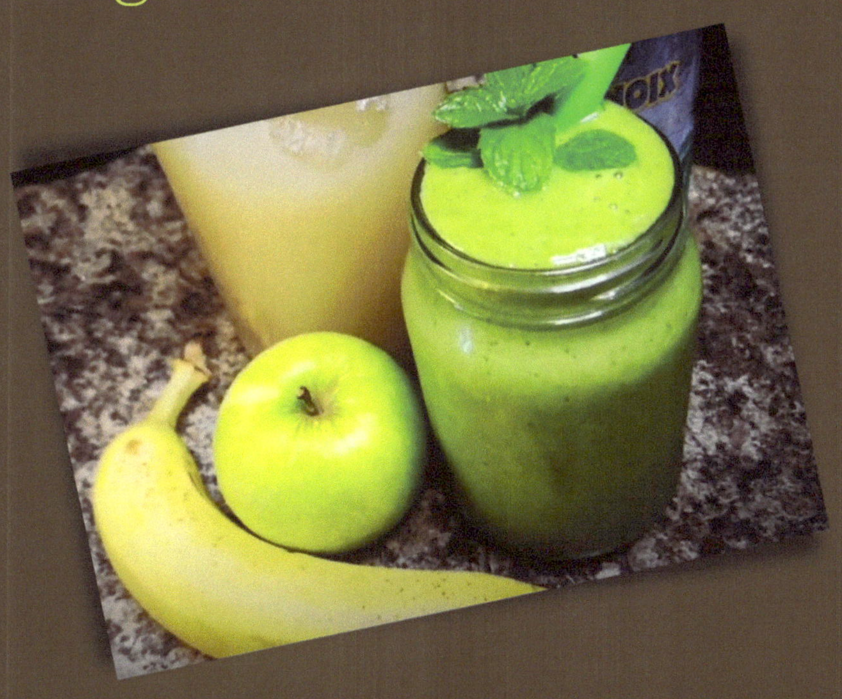

CAN YOU EAT TOO MUCH SEA MOSS?

It doesn't take much to start out adding **Sea moss** into your diet, so a serving of **Sea moss** is simply two tablespoons. **Sea moss** is a source of iodine, which is something you can eat an excessive amount of.

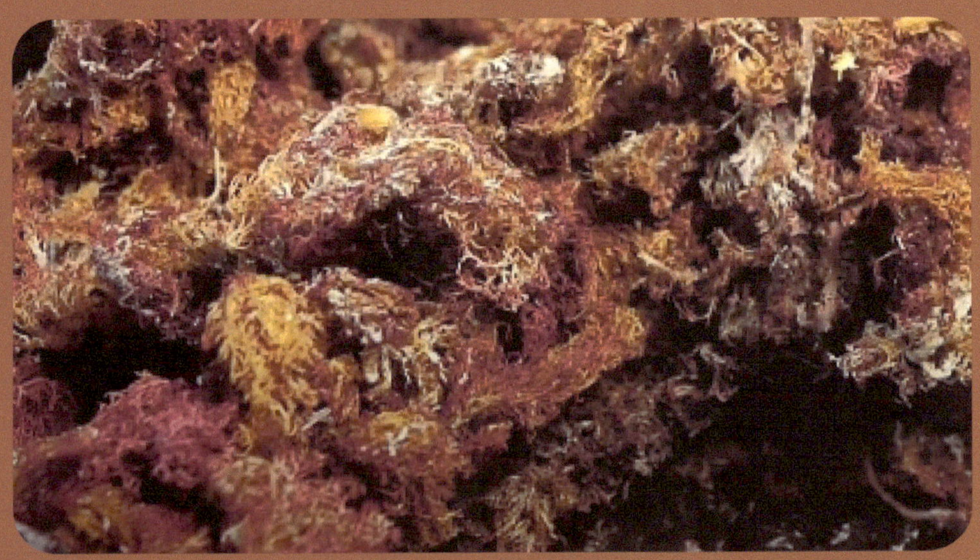

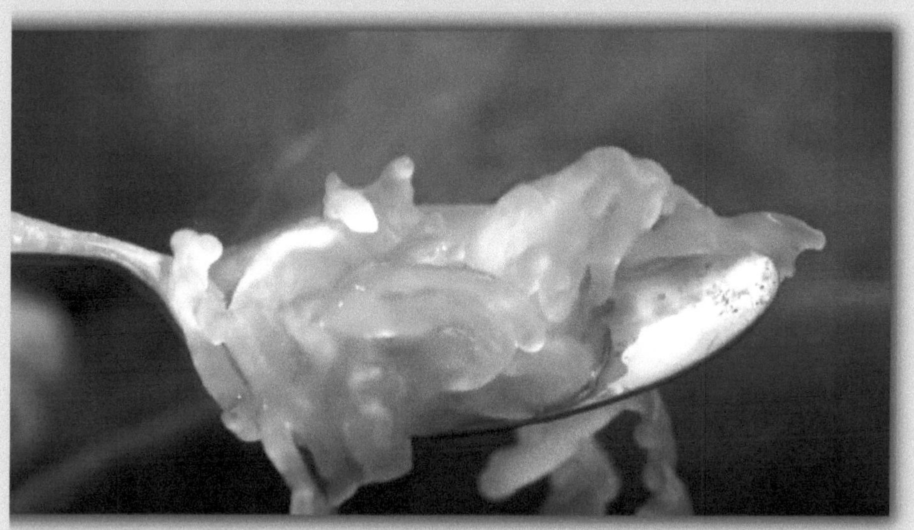

DIGESTIVE AID

Sea moss also has anti-inflammatory properties, which may be great for soothing the gut. The lining of probiotics act as a lubricant, making it easier for waste to move through your bowels. The good is...be ready to pass waste easily and frequently without straining.

WHAT IS THE BEST WAY TO CONSUME SEA MOSS?

The best way by far to enjoy the benefits of **Sea moss** is to put it in a smoothie drink. Because sea moss has a light taste it will be masked by whatever fruits and vegetables you decide to use.

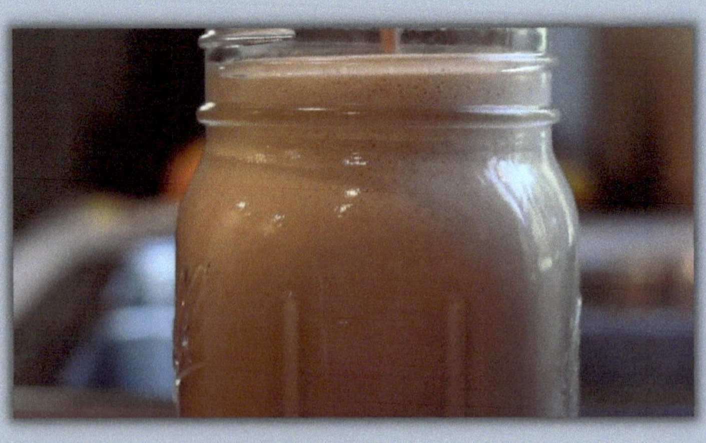

CAN SEA MOSS GEL GO BAD?

Sea moss is a natural product made from organic matter (seaweed) it is going to deteriorate over time.A batch will last you up 3 weeks.

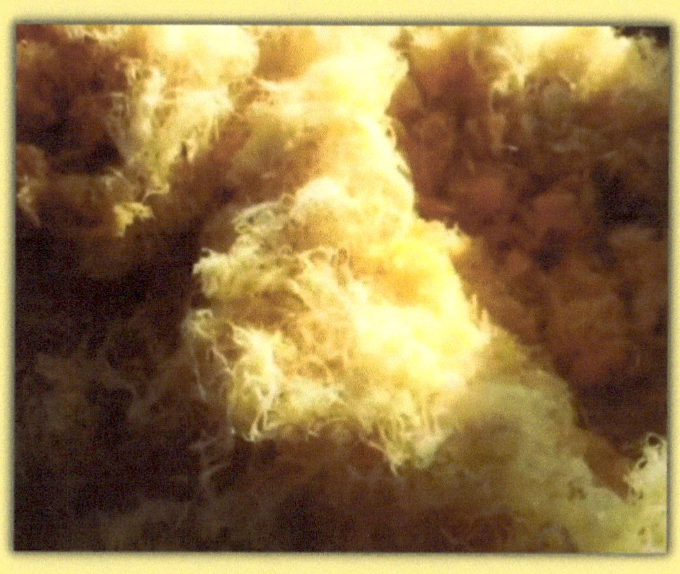

BLADDERWRACK

WHAT IS BLADDERWRACK GOOD FOR?

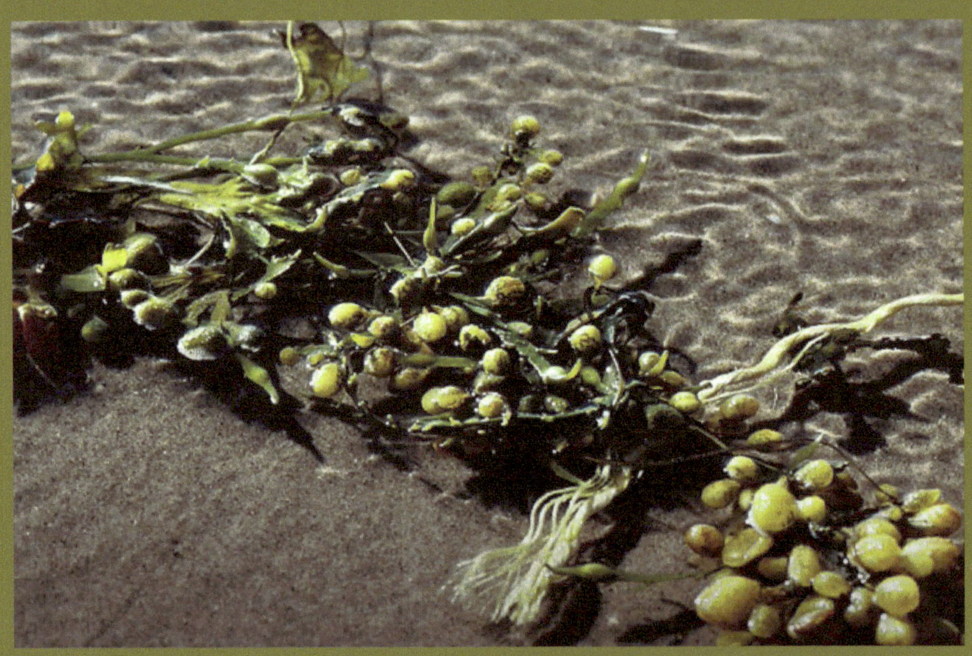

Bladderwrack is used to treat obesity, arthritis, joint pain, "hardening of the arteries" (arteriosclerosis), digestive disorders, heartburn, "blood cleansing," constipation, bronchitis, emphysema, urinary tract disorders, and anxiety. Other uses include boosting the immune system and increasing energy.

SHOULD I TAKE BLADDERWRACK?

You should consult a doctor before using **Bladderwrack**. Pregnant or breastfeeding women should not take **Bladderwrack**. It is one of the highest iodine-containing sea vegetables or plants known to man.

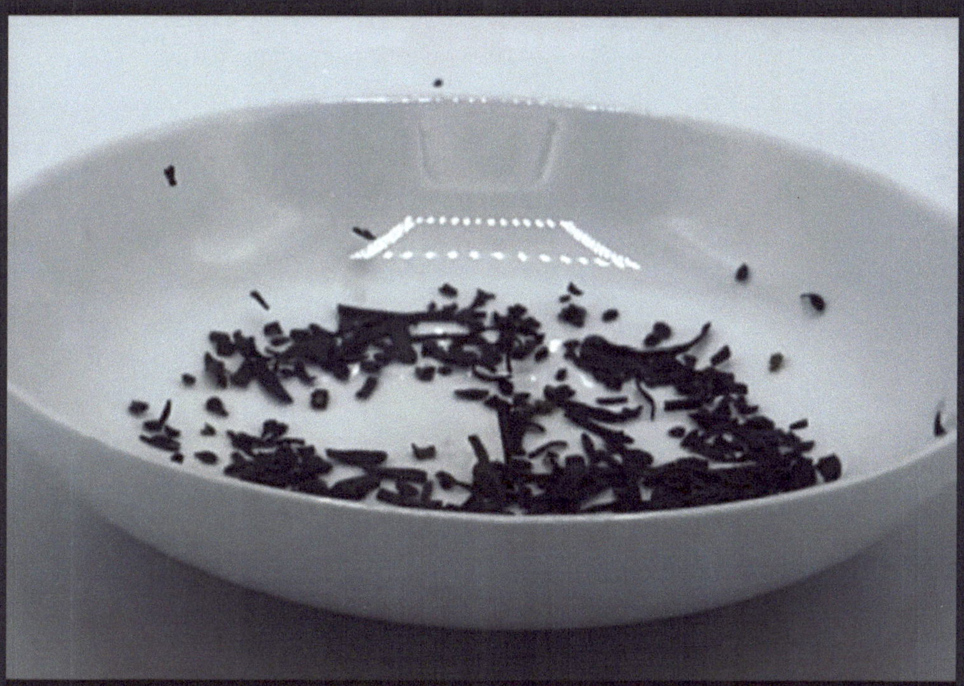

ARE THERE ANY SIDE EFFECTS?

Bladderwrack can cause acne, thyroid dysfunction, and heavy-metal contamination. Any form of Iodine, including **Bladderwrack** and other seaweeds—can cause or aggravate acne in some people. Other side effects are upset stomach, changes in urination, bleeding, rash, high blood pressure, menstruation, angioedema, fever, and arthralgia.

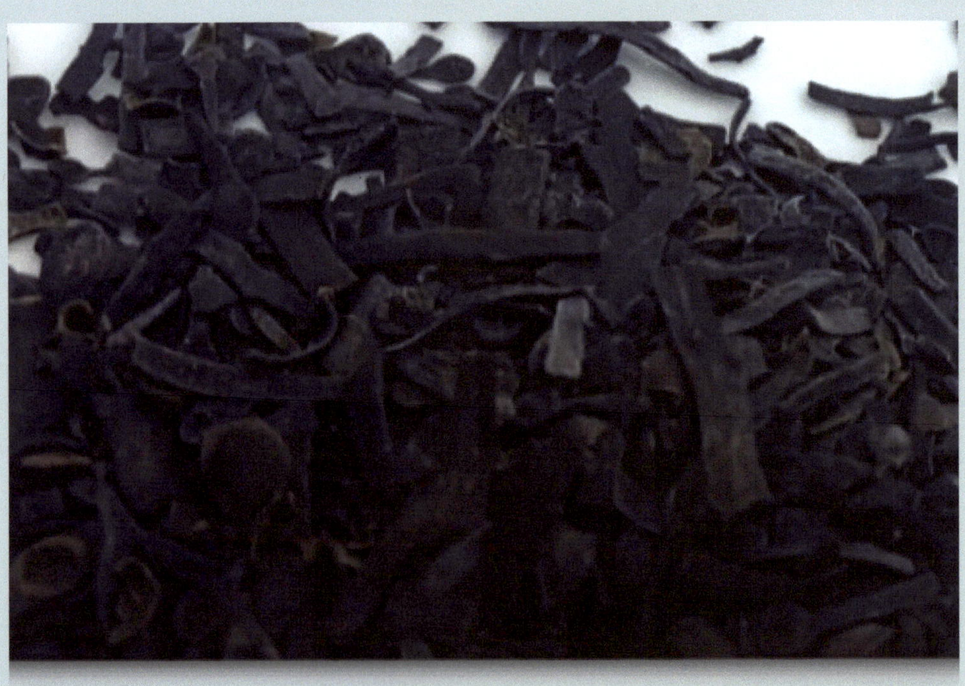

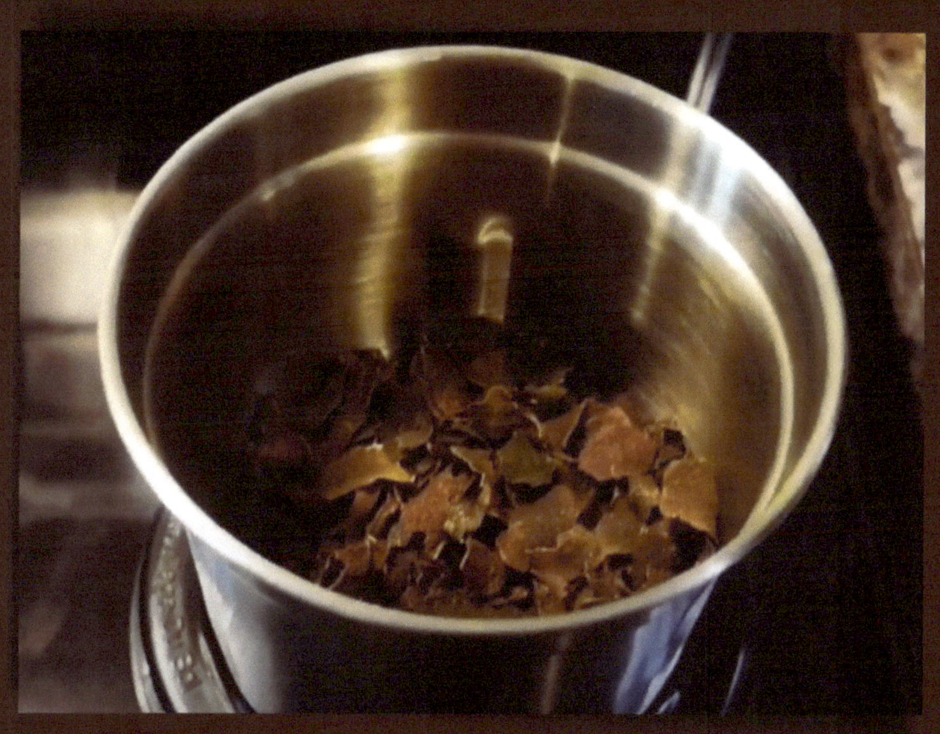

CAN I TAKE BLADDERWRACK EVERYDAY?

It's better to limit your intake to no more than 2 cups (500 mL) per day to avoid consuming too much iodine and other active ingredients in **Bladderwrack**. You can purchase it dried, powdered, as a dietary supplement, or in the form of tea.

CAN BLADDERWRACK CAUSE HEADACHE?

Bladderwrack can cause unexplained weight loss, fast heartbeat, or shakiness. You may experience very bad headaches, high blood pressure, nervousness, problems breathing, or nosebleeds

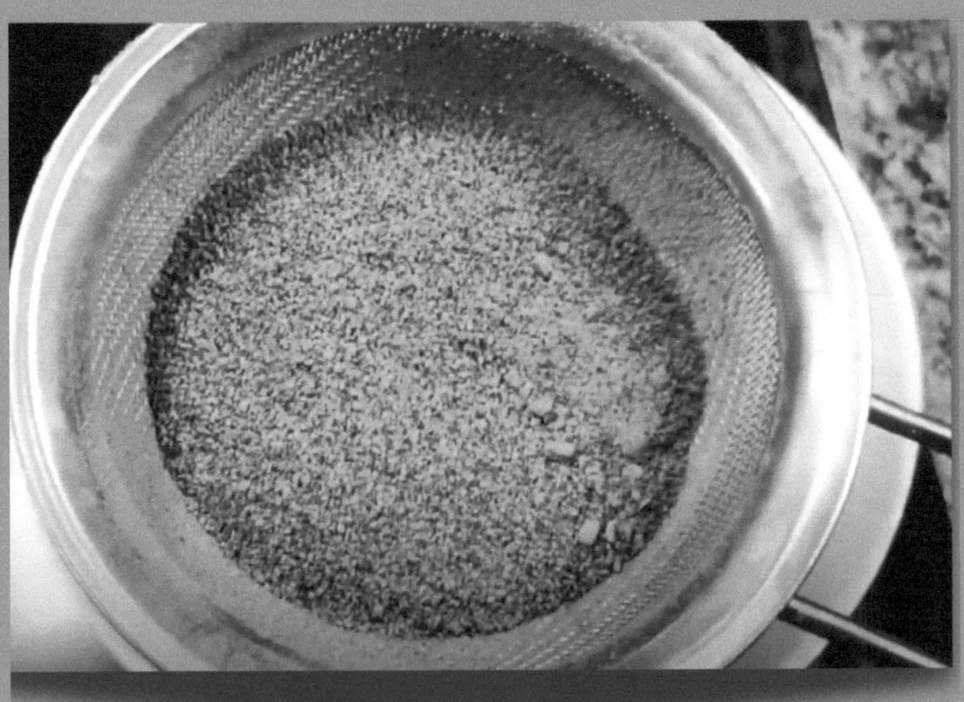

BURDOCK ROOTS

NATIVE TO EUROPE AND NORTHERN ASIA, **BURDOCK ROOT** IS A VEGETABLE THAT GROWS IN THE UNITED STATES. THE **BURDOCK PLANT** HAS DEEP AND VERY LONG ROOTS THAT VARY IN COLOR FROM BEIGE TO BROWN AND NEARLY BLACK ON THE OUTSIDE.

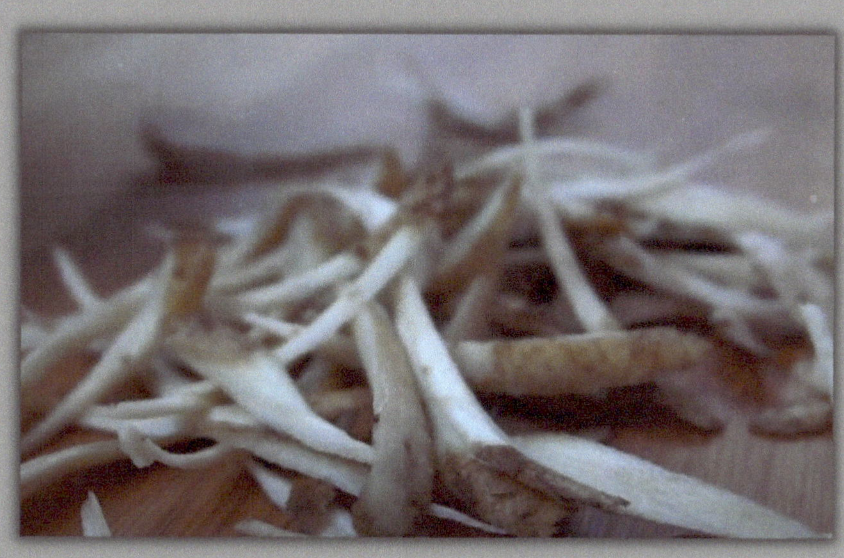

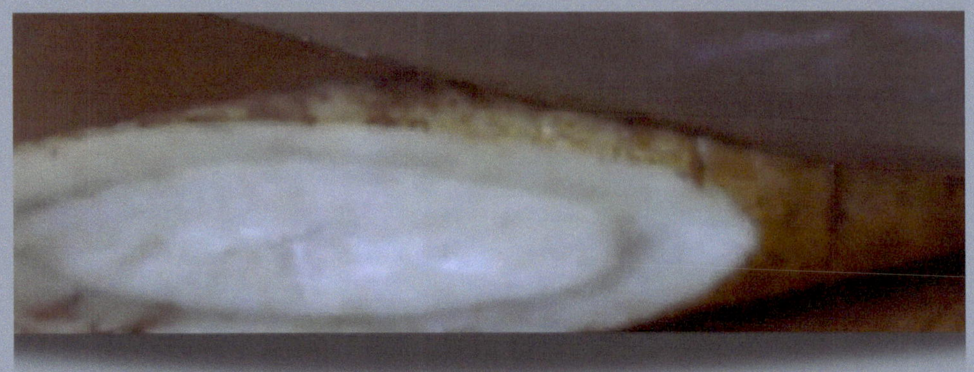

DOES BURDOCK ROOT CLEANSE THE LIVER?

Burdock root enhances elimination by way of the liver, as it is mildly a laxative. It is helpful for a 'sluggish' liver with feelings of fullness, chronic constipation, and poor fat digestion. **Burdock root** is a gentle herb that improves liver function and elimination.

WHAT IS BURDOCK TEA GOOD FOR?

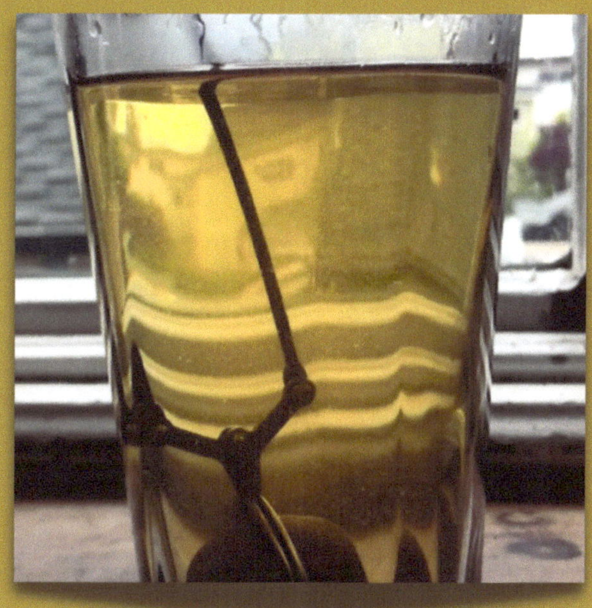

Burdock Tea is used to increase urine flow, kill germs, reduce fever, and "purify" your blood. It can also be used to treat colds, cancer, anorexia nervosa, gastrointestinal (GI) complaints, joint pain (rheumatism), gout, bladder infections, complications of syphilis, and skin conditions including acne and psoriasis.

WHAT ARE THE SIDE EFFECTS OF BURDOCK ROOT?

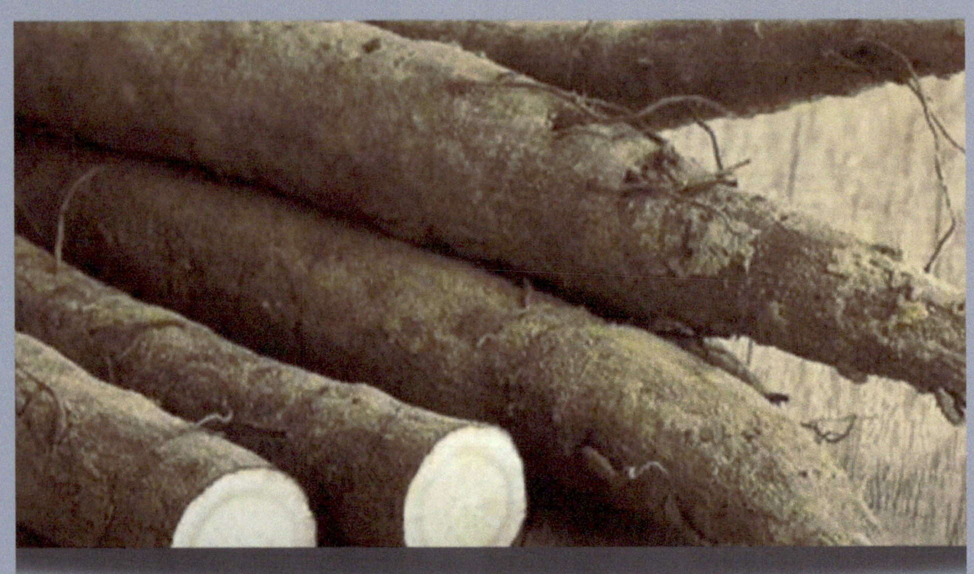

For some people, **Burdock Tea** might slow blood clotting. People with bleeding disorders risk of bleeding might increase. People who are allergic to ragweed and related plants may experience a reaction, this includes people who are sensitive to the Asteraceae/Compositae family.

IS BURDOCK ROOT GOOD FOR YOUR HAIR?

Regular use of **Burdock Root** in hair care has been shown to promote healthy hair growth, soothe inflammation and scalp conditions, and leave hair soft, smooth and shiny. The extract in burdock is beneficial for all hair types.

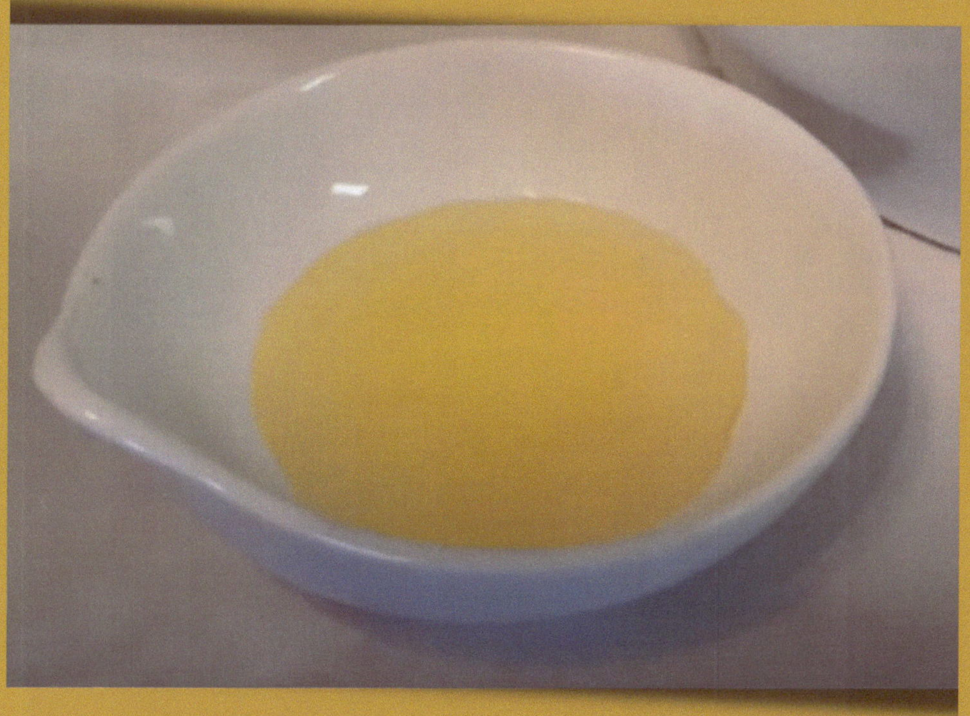

HOW MUCH BURDOCK ROOT SHOULD I TAKE DAILY?

Dosages used in studies vary up to six grams a day of **Burdock root** tea, the minimum being from 200 milligrams of burdock root extract. Patients with advanced refractory pancreatic cancer are recommended 12 grams a day.

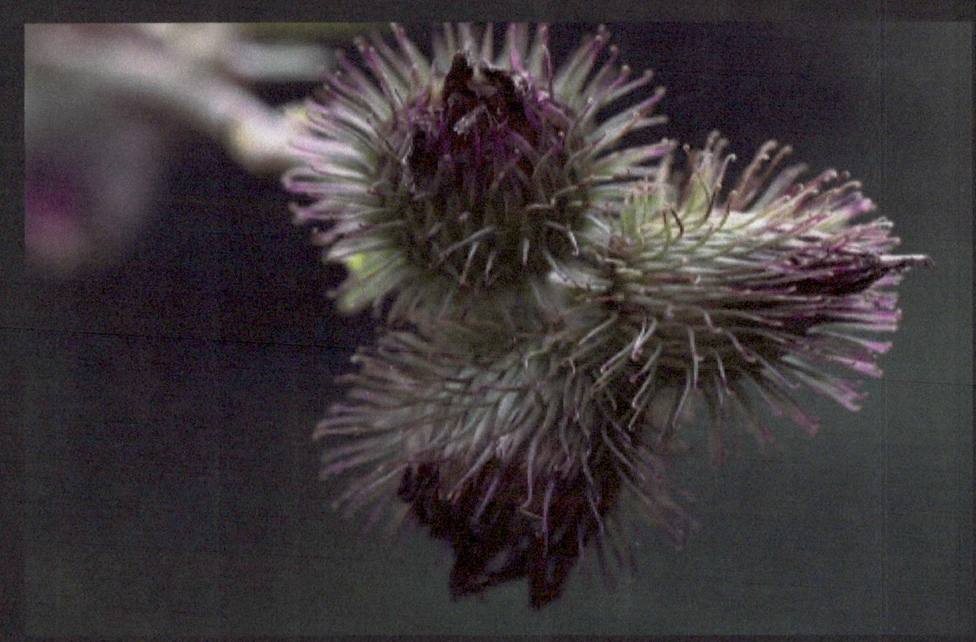

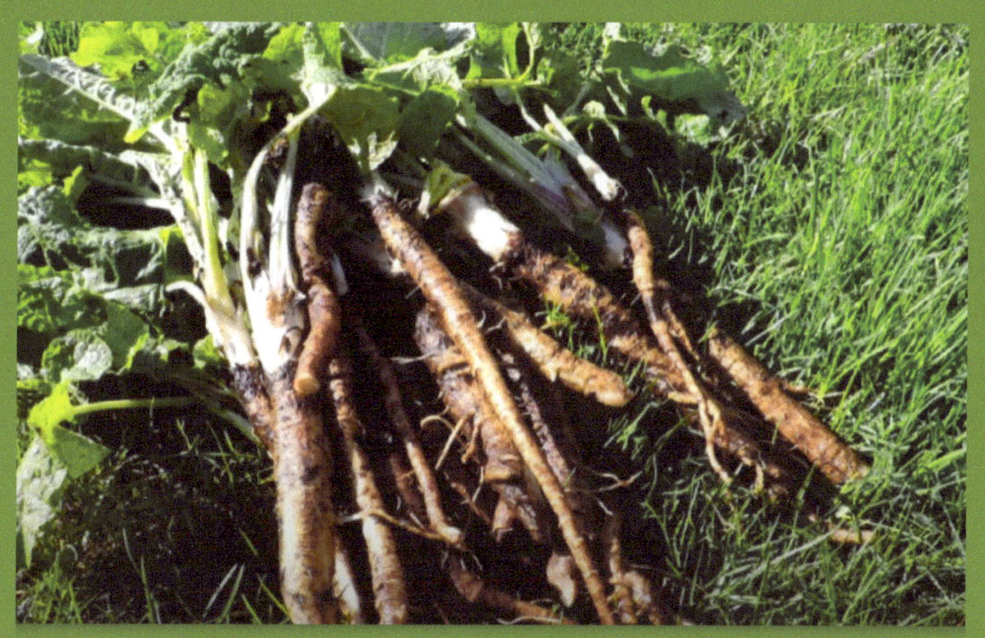

WHO SHOULD NOT TAKE BURDOCK ROOT?

Women who are pregnant, want to become pregnant, or who are breastfeeding should not take **Burdock Root**. Children under 18 and people with a history of allergies to plants, should not take unless a doctor suggests otherwise.

DOES BURDOCK ROOT GIVE YOU ENERGY?

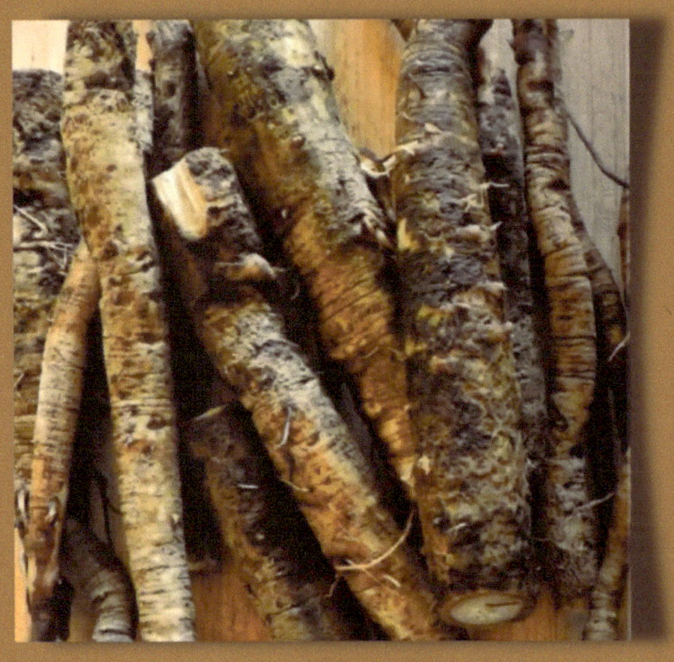

Burdock needs to be used with commitment over several months a few doses won't do the trick.

Burdock will show you its ability to nourish depleted bodies, provide increased energy, and improve the function of the digestive system over time.

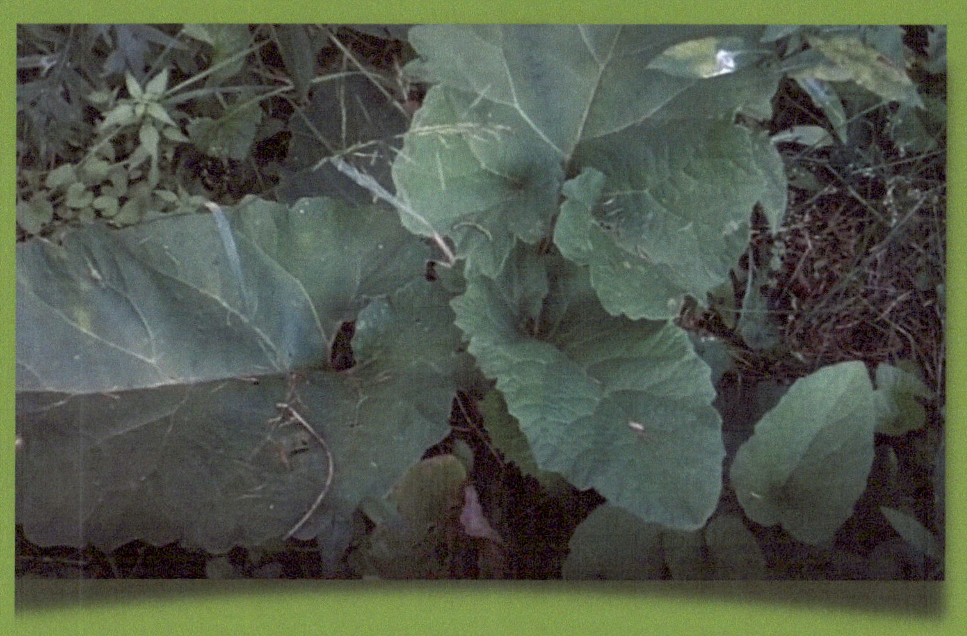

WHAT PARTS OF BURDOCK ARE EDIBLE?

The young central stalk, which is only available for a short time in the early summer. The petioles or leaf stalks are a great deal of work to prepare, but have a longer season, and the root is also edible.

OIL OF OREGANO

WHAT ARE THE BENEFITS OF OIL OF OREGANO?

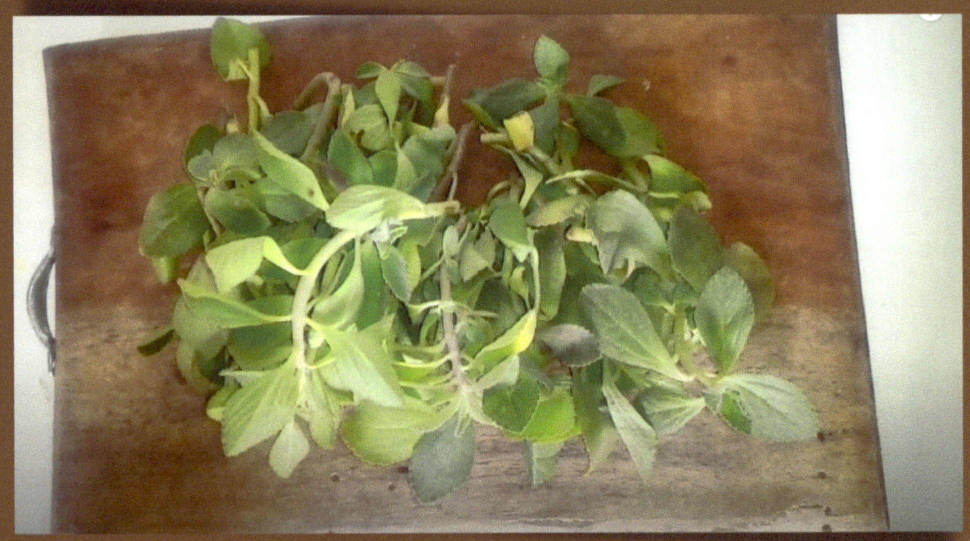

Oregano oil is a natural antibiotic, it may help lower cholesterol, it's a powerful anti-oxidant and it could help treat yeast infections. **Oregano oil** can improve gut health. It also has anti-inflammatory properties also help relieve pain, and it has some cancer-fighting properties.

CAN I TAKE OIL OF OREGANO DAILY?

It's easy to take too much **Oil of Oregano** or to use it for too long. Unlike the herb you cook with, **Oil of Oregano** commercially prepared is highly concentrated. **Oil of Oregano** when used as directed should be safe. It may have detrimental effects in too-high doses.

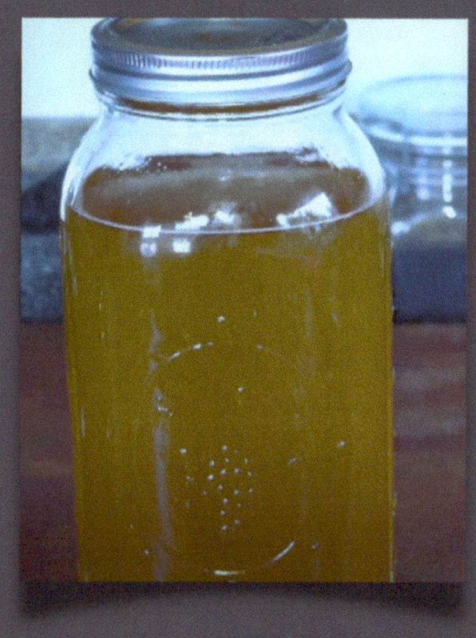

CAN OREGANO CURE COUGH?

The chemicals **Oregano** contains might help reduce cough and spasms. Oregano increases bile flow aiding digestion and fighting against some bacteria, viruses, fungi, intestinal worms, and other parasites.

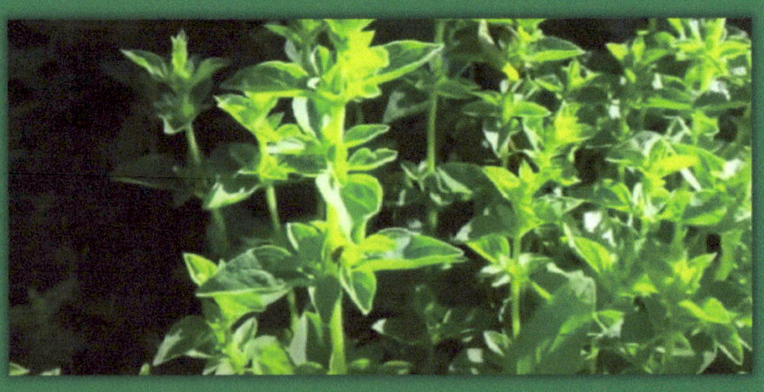

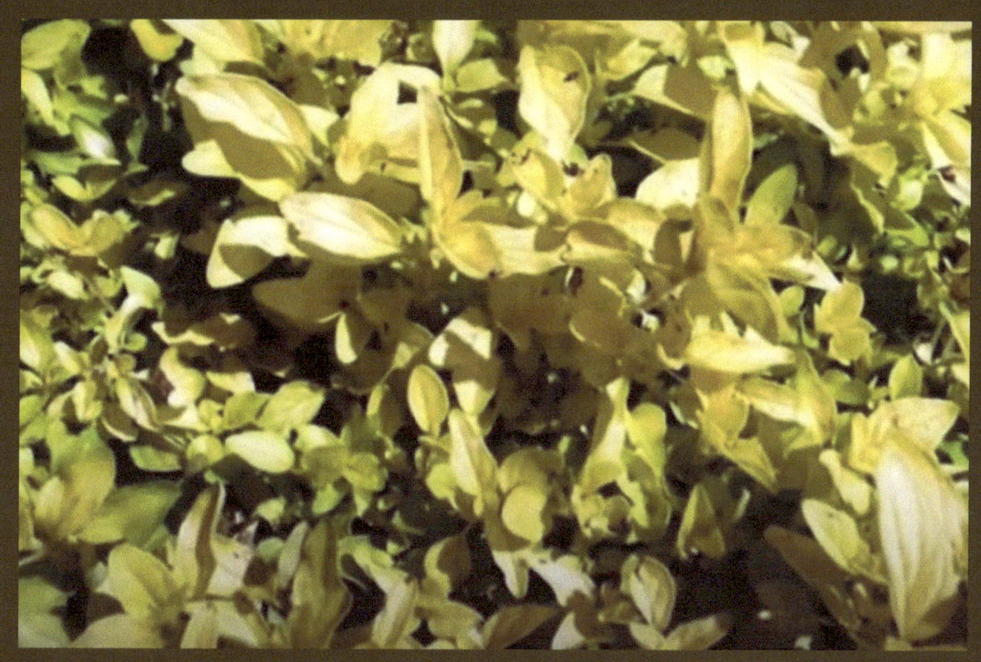

DOES OIL OF OREGANO KILL GOOD BACTERIA?

Research shows **Oregano Oil** is effective against strains of bacteria, including E.coli and Pseudomonas aeruginosa. It's best mixed with water or coconut oil.

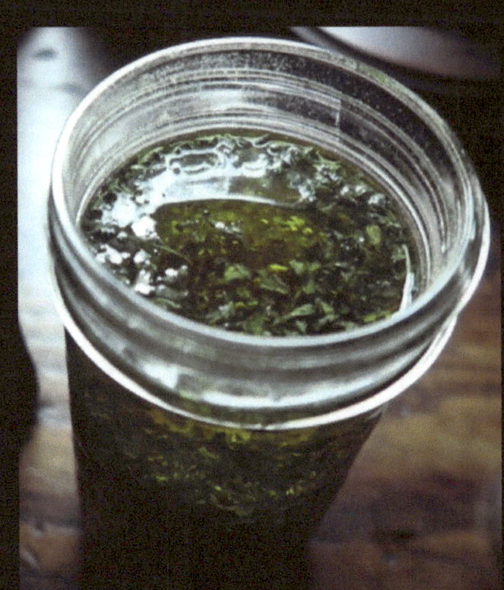

DOES OREGANO OIL KILL WARTS?

Oregano oil has properties that make it helpful for treating warts. It contains compounds that give it antifungal, antioxidant, anti-inflammatory and pain-killing properties. It also contains carvacrol, which has been researched for its antiviral properties.

DOES OIL OF OREGANO LOWER BLOOD PRESSURE?

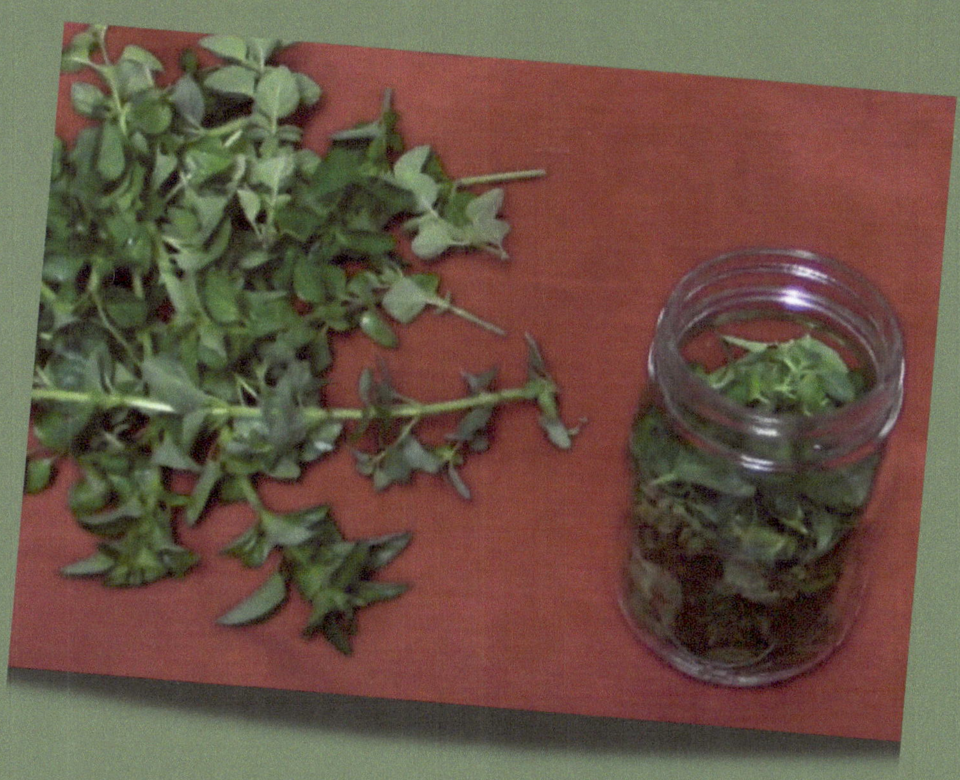

Oil of Oregano helps prevent many bacterial, viral, and fungal infections. It also helps high blood pressure, digestion and calms the nerves.

DOES OREGANO OIL INTERACT WITH ANY MEDICATIONS?

Taking oregano along with medications that slow clotting might increase the chances of bruising and bleeding in theory. Medications that slow blood clotting include aspirin, Plavix, Pradaxa, Fragmin, Lovenox, heparin, Coumadin, and others.

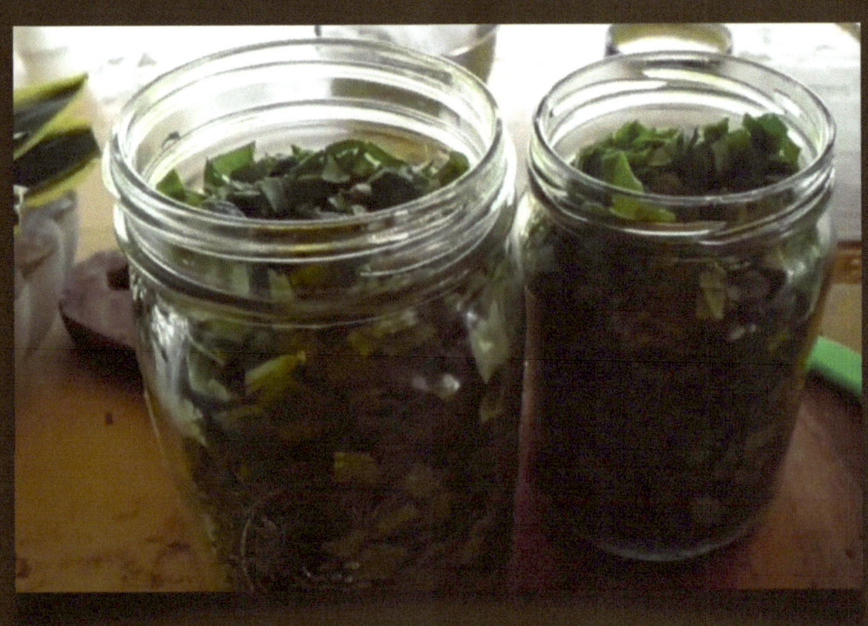

CAN I TAKE OREGANO OIL INTERNALLY?

Oregano oil can be taken internally only if it's 100 percent therapeutic grade oil. ... Before using oregano essential oil on your skin, always mix it with coconut oil or jojoba oil. This will help to reduce the risk of irritation and adverse reactions

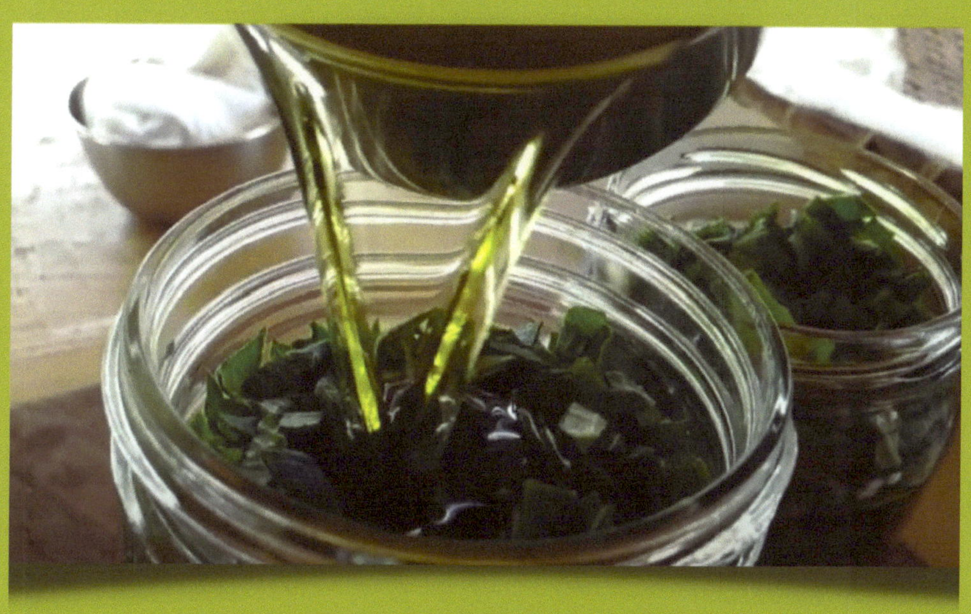

A few drops of Oregano oil on affected nails twice daily can help dissolve the diseased portion of a nail, leaving the healthy part intact.

DOES OREGANO OIL KILL TOENAIL FUNGUS?

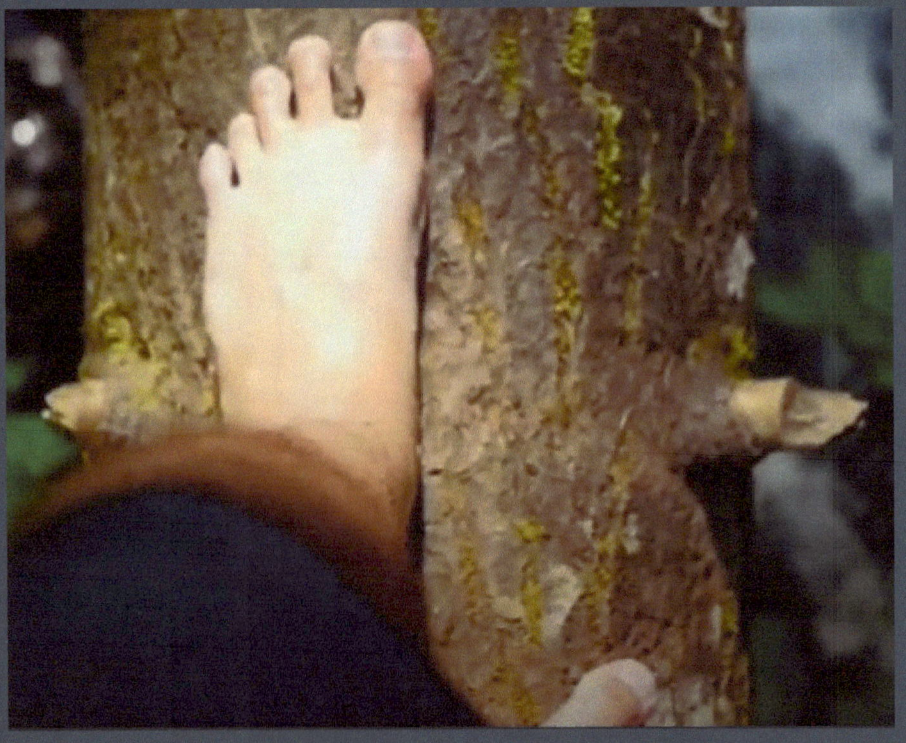

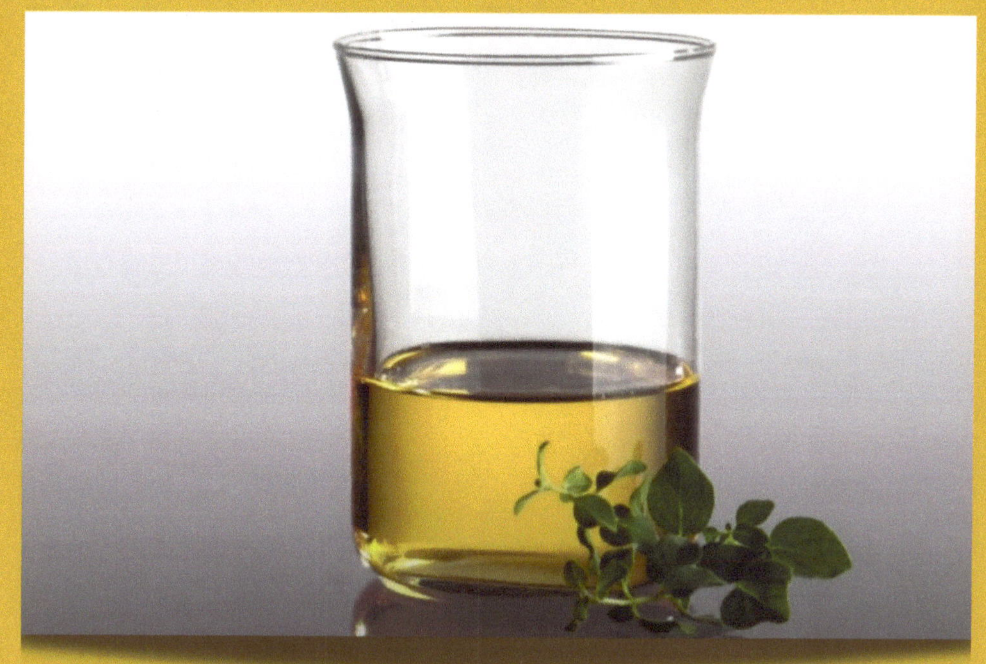

OREGANO OIL FOR YEAST INFECTION?

Oil of Oregano can be applied to a tampon before insertion. Alternately capsules containing it may be inserted into the vagina at night. **Oil of Oregano** was in some studies to inhibit the growth of candida.

MULLEIN LEAF

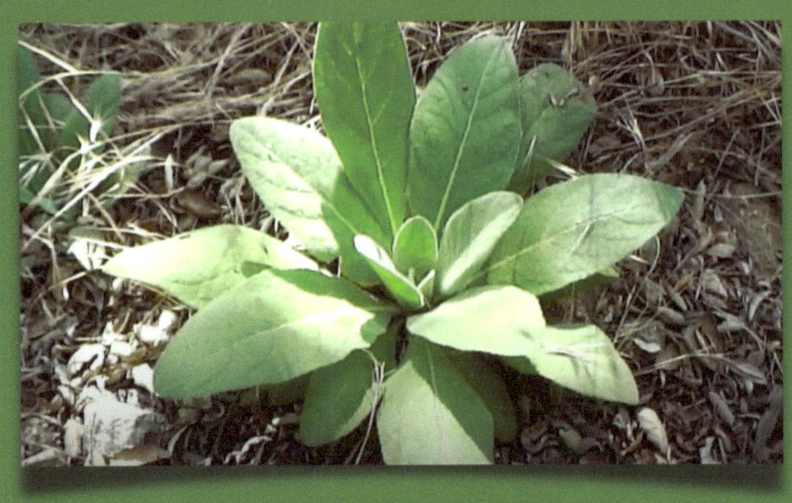

Recent studies show that **Mullein** is used for cough, whooping cough, tuberculosis, bronchitis, hoarseness, pneumonia, earaches, colds, chills, flu, swine flu, fever, allergies, tonsillitis, and sore throat. Other uses include asthma, diarrhea, colic, gastrointestinal bleeding, migraines, joint pain, and gout.

IS MULLEIN GOOD FOR THE LUNGS?

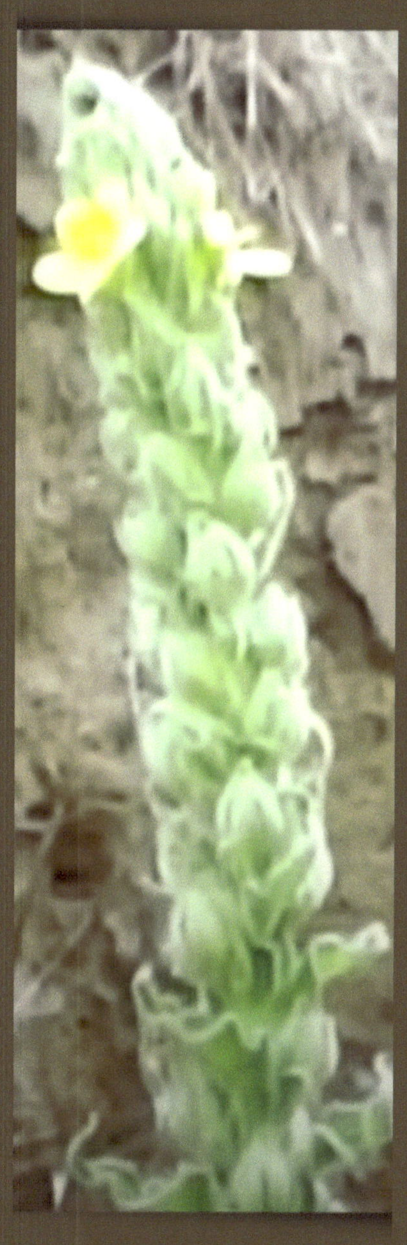

Mullein helps ease spasms, tightness, cough, open the lungs, and soothes irritation and dryness. It is a safe, and profound respiratory tonic.

SIDE EFFECTS OF MULLEIN?

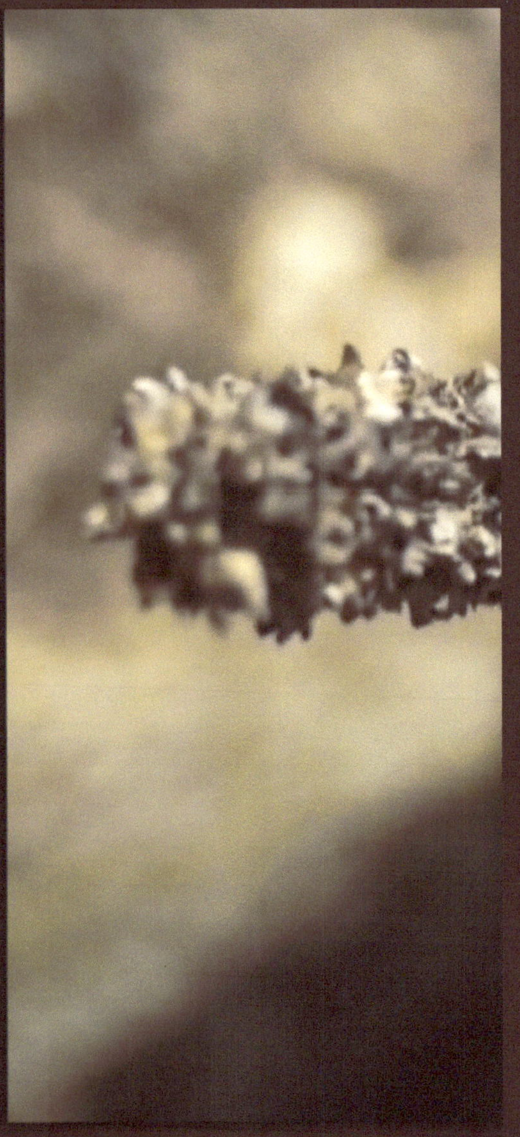

Some species of **Mullein** may cause itching, rash, and irritation. Be sure to do a patch skin test before using **Mullein** on your skin.

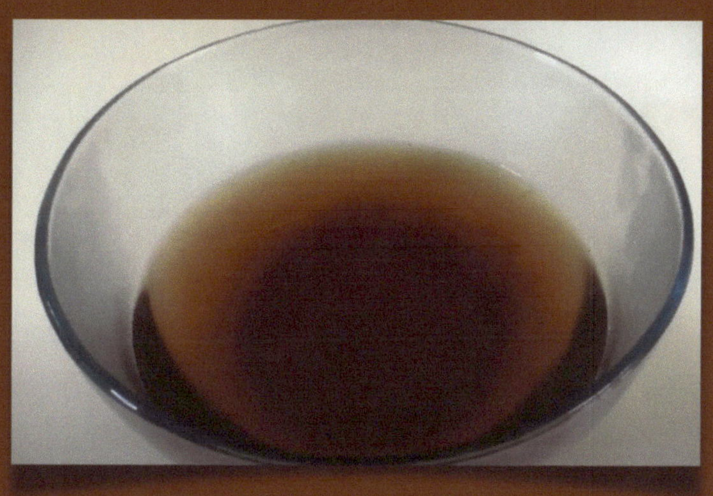

IS MULLEIN TEA SAFE TO DRINK?

Mullein tea should be strained properly and exercise caution if handling the herb directly to prevent skin irritation. It is considered to besafe and has few side effects.

IS MULLEIN GOOD FOR MUCUS?

Mullein is classified as a expectorant in herbal literature. Mullein promotes the discharge of mucus, and a demulcent, to soothe and protect mucous membranes.

IS MULLEIN TOXIC?

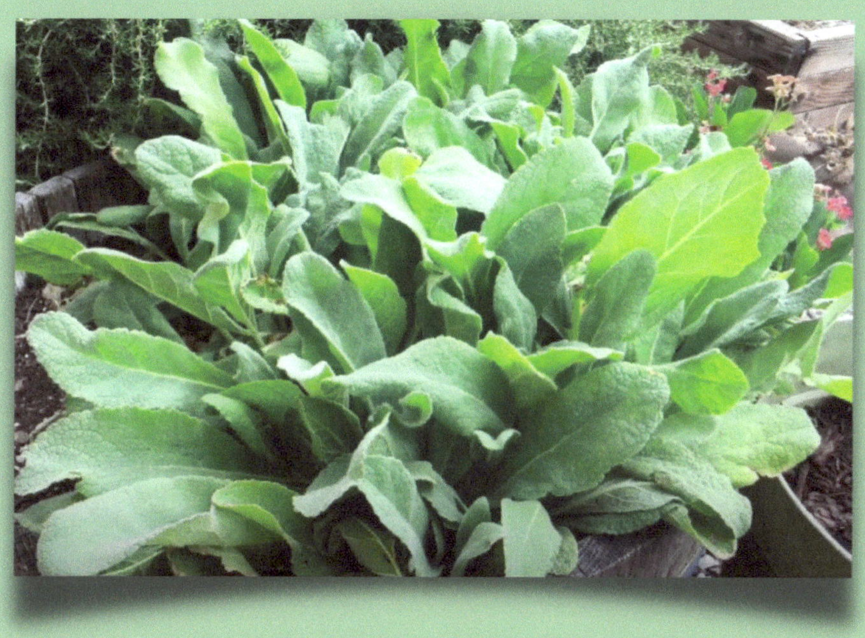

There has not been any credible reports of serious adverse effects. However, **Mullein** seeds do contain the insecticide and fish poison Rotenone, which is relatively safe in humans, it does however present some toxic risks. **Mullein leaves** and flowers are on the FDA's GRAS list.

WHAT IS ELDERBERRY GOOD FOR?

Elderberries are packed with antioxidants and vitamins that boost the immune system. Some benefits are that it helps tame inflammation, lessen stress, and protect the heart. Other benefits include preventing and the easing cold and flu symptoms.

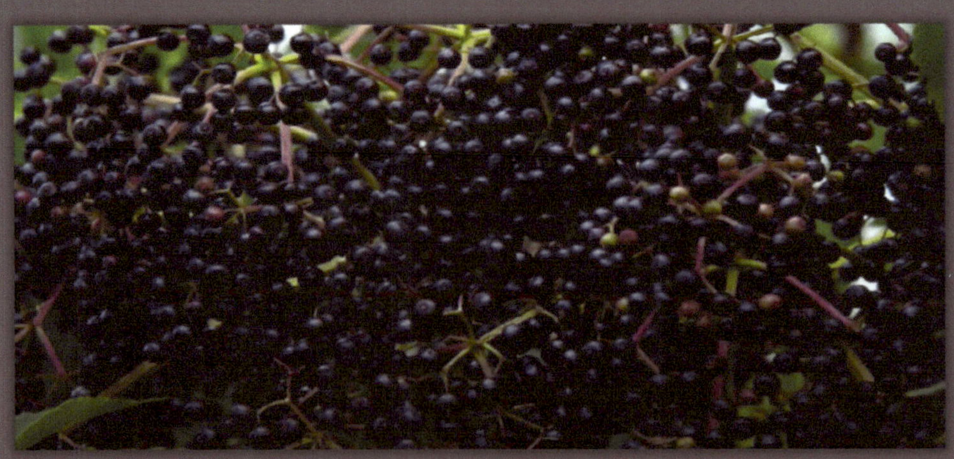

IS IT OK TO TAKE ELDERBERRY EVERYDAY?

It's best to never eat or drink any product made from raw elderberry fruit, flowers, or leaves. **Elderberry** when used daily for up to five days has low risks. The safety of its long-term use is not yet confirmed.

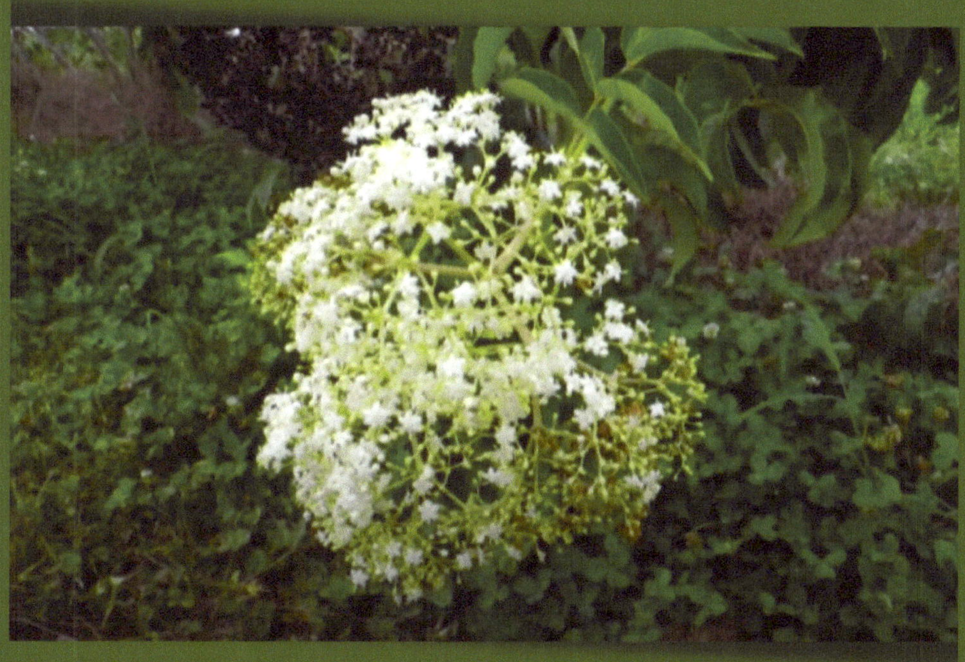

ARE ELDERBERRIES SAFE TO EAT?

The blue or purple **Elderberries** are gathered and made into wine, jam, syrup, and pies. You can eat the petals raw or make a fragrant and tasty tea.

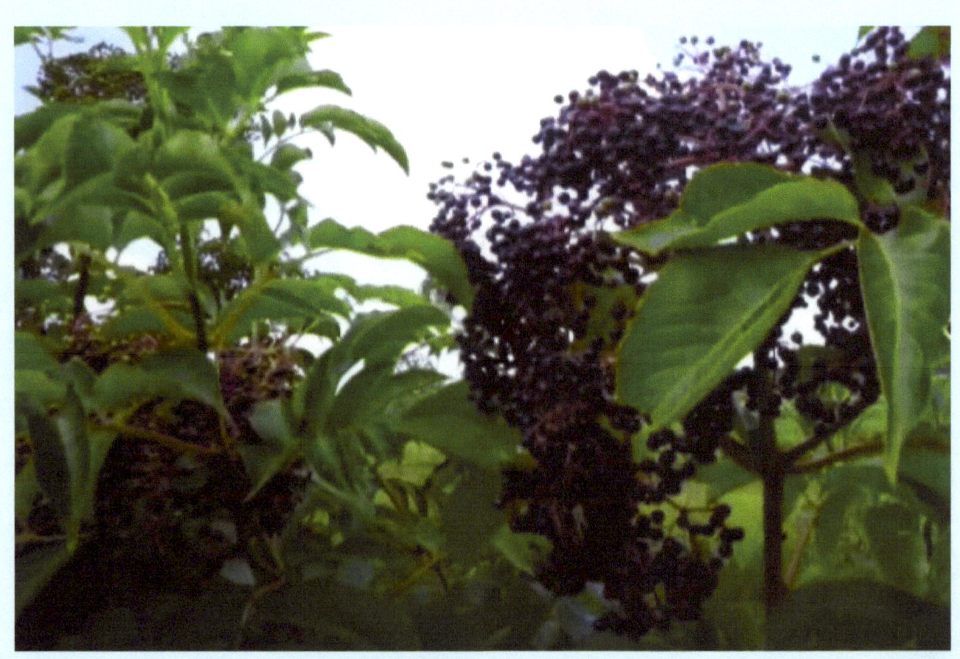

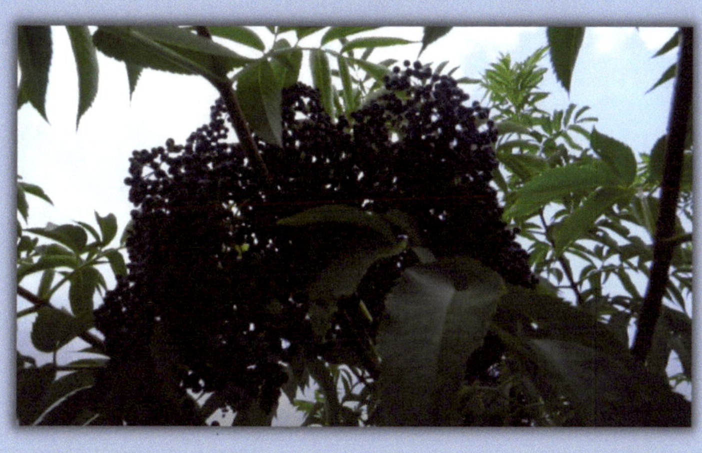

IS ELDERBERRY GOOD FOR WEIGHT LOSS?

Elderberry is among the top sources of antioxidants, which play a proven role in reducing inflammation. One dose of elderberry may help keep you on track with your fitness and weight loss goals.

WHO SHOULD NOT USE ELDERBERRY SYRUP?

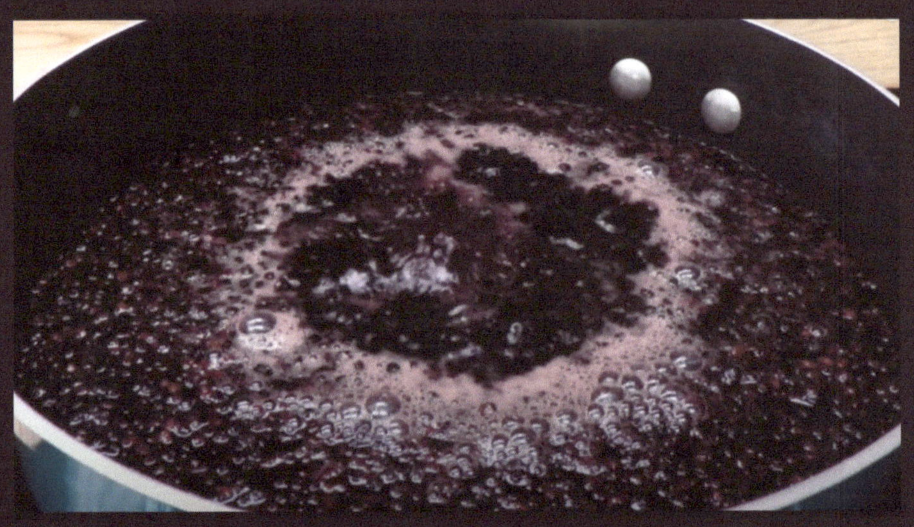

Elderberry is not recommended for children and adolescents under 18 years of age or pregnant or lactating women. There have not been any adverse reports in these groups, but there is also not enough data to confirm that it is safe. Be sure to remove any bark or leaves before use.

DOES ELDERBERRY AFFECT THYROID?

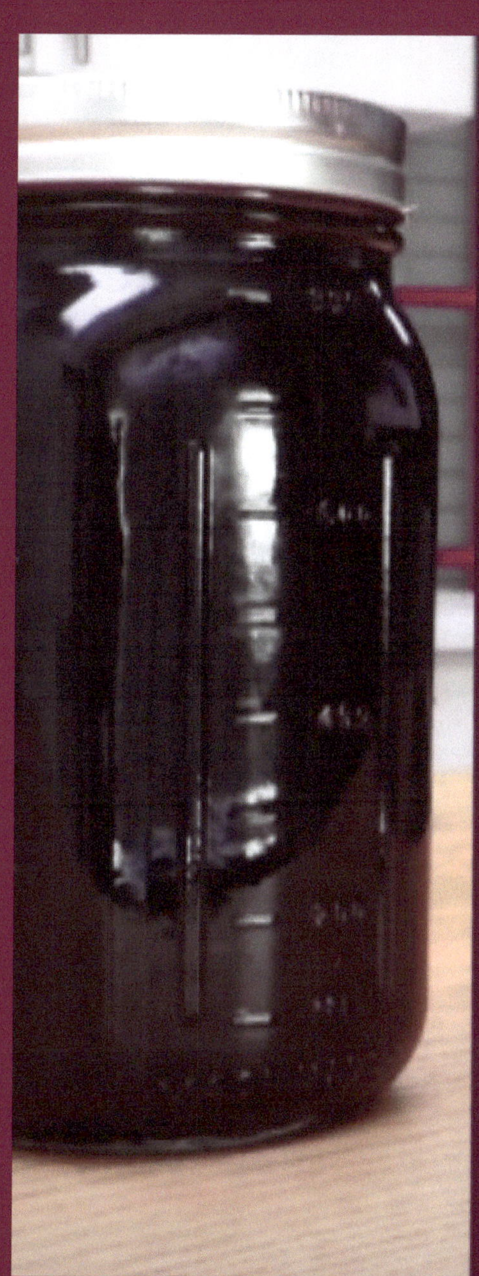

Elderberry may be detrimental for people with autoimmune disorders. Elderberry may cause more damage and inflammation to the thyroid gland by supporting the immune cells that specifically attack your thyroid gland.

DOES ELDERBERRY INTERACT WITH MEDICATIONS?

Elderberry can increase the immune system, but taking elderberry along with some medications that decrease the immune system might decrease the effectiveness of medications that decrease the immune system.

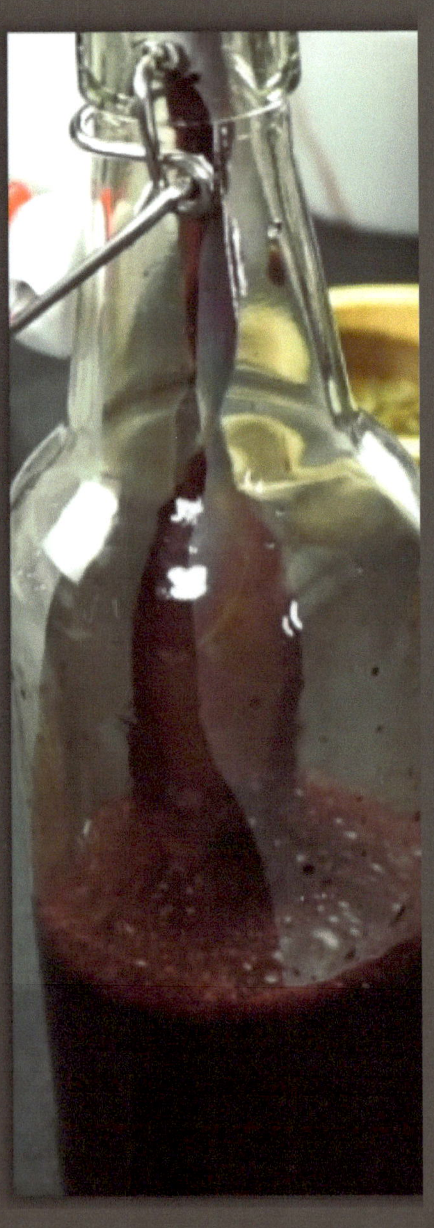

IS ELDERBERRY GOOD FOR SKIN?

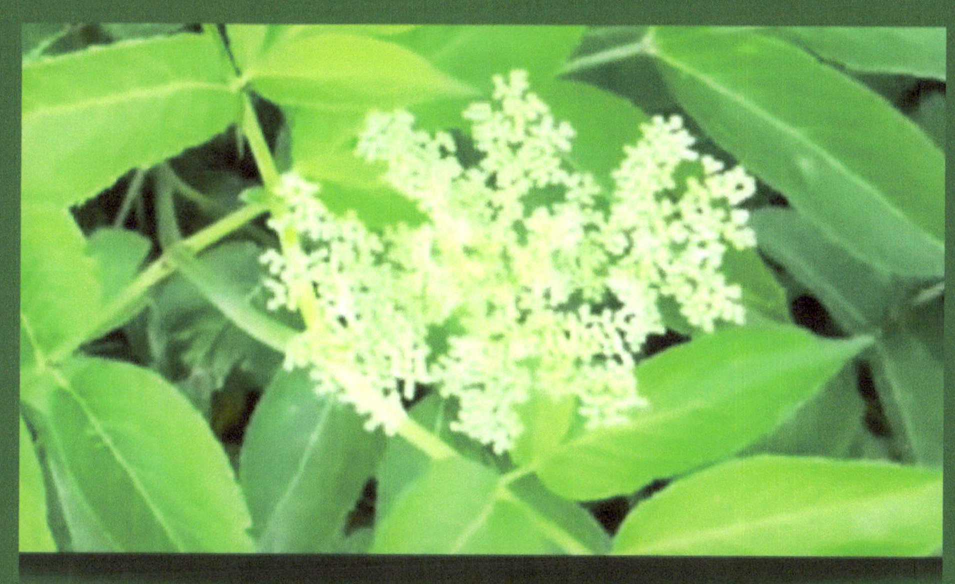

Elderberries are infused with anti-aging and free-radical fighting properties, the elderberries keep your skin radiant and healthy. Elderberry also helps keep away distressing skin conditions like breakouts, boils, and scars.

IS ELDERBERRY GOOD FOR INFLAMMATION?

Elderberries have remarkable antioxidant and anti-inflammatory effects. Research has supported the anti-inflammatory and antioxidant effects of elderberry. Elderberry has been a staple in natural medicine for hundreds of years.

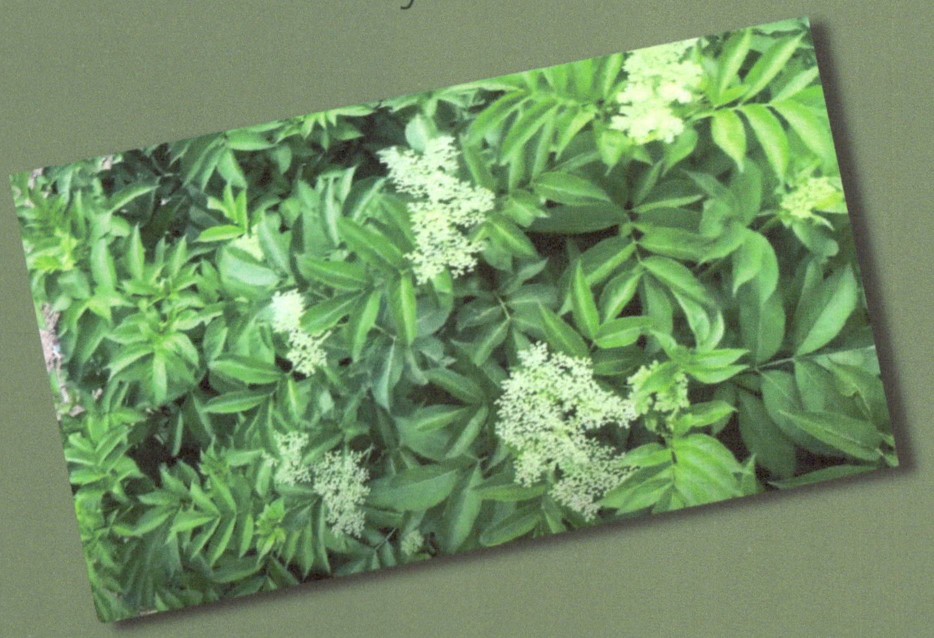

JAMAICAN SARSPARILLA ROOT

Sarsaparilla root is known for its medicinal benefits. It is very high in iron and it's good for people dealing with anemia.

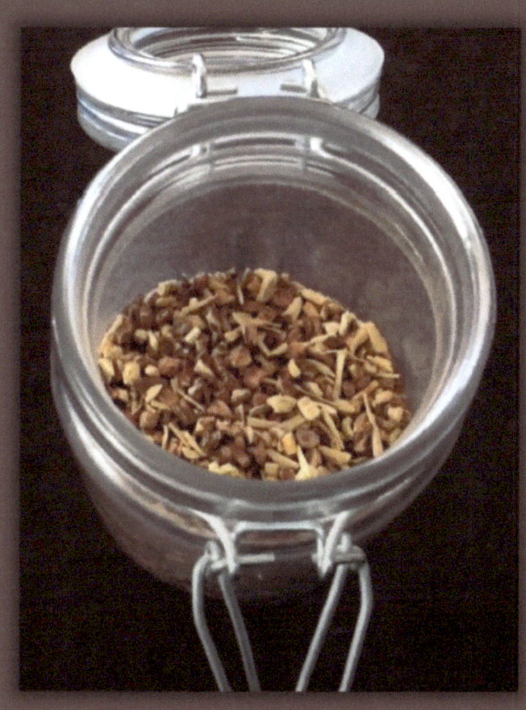

WHO IS SARSAPARILLA BAD FOR?

People suffering from Asthma may experience a runny nose. **Sarsaparilla** might make kidney disease worse. Avoid **Sarsaparilla** if you have kidney problems.

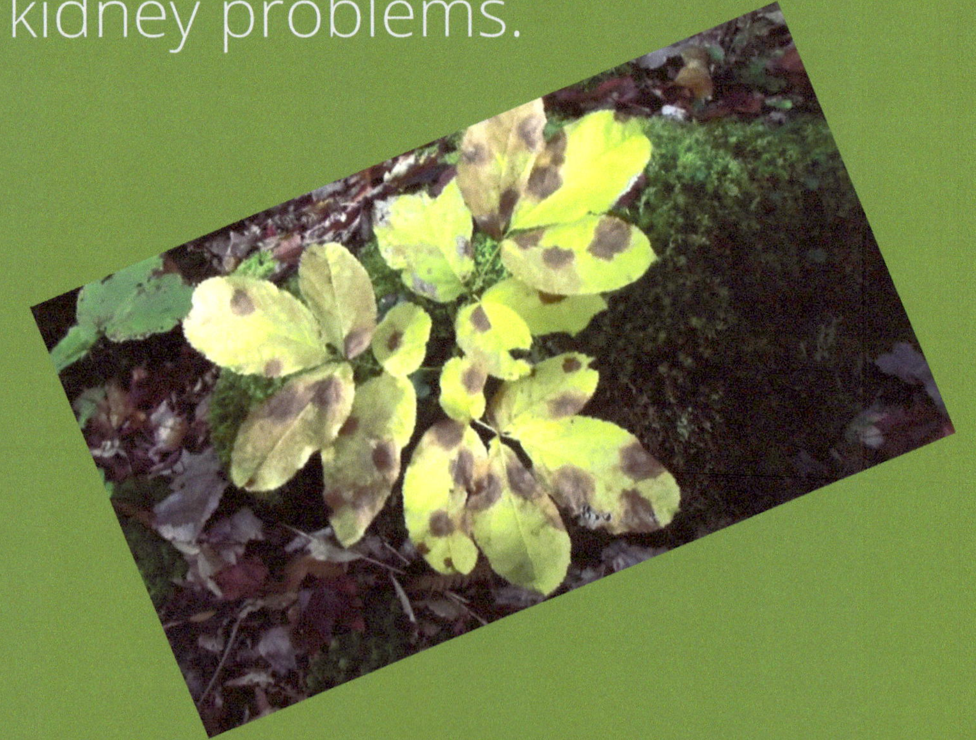

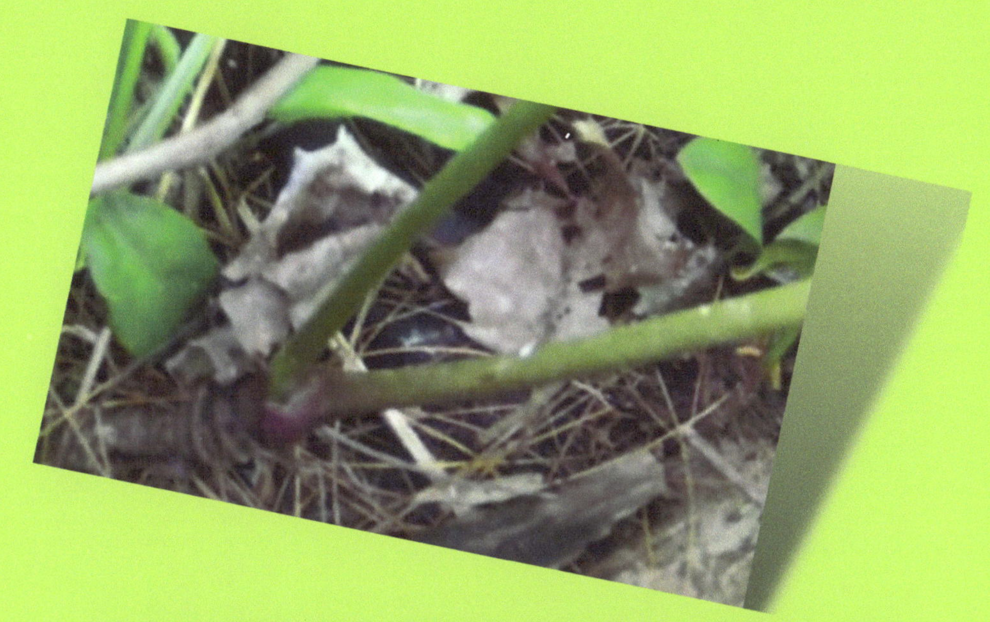

WHAT IS SARSAPARILLA ROOT GOOD FOR?

Sarsaparilla root has been used for centuries around the world. The root of the plant has been used to treat joint problems like arthritis, and for healing skin problems like psoriasis, eczema, and dermatitis. The root has been thought to cure leprosy because of its "blood-purifying" properties.